WORK WITH IT!

MY HAIR GROWTH STORY

Simple steps towards growing Healthy Afro Hair

Julie Oli

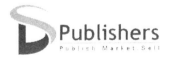

Publishers
Publish Market Sell

For permission request, contact the publisher
at the email address below:
Email: info@sdpublishers.com
Website: www.sdpublishers.com

Author: Julie Oli
Publisher: SDPublishers

Cover Design: Joanne Oli
Cover Image: Andrew Irabor
Typeset: SDPublishers Design Unit

Distributed by SDPublishers

Paperback ISBN: 978-1-908386-05-2

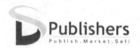

Acknowledgments

Firstly, I'd like to take this opportunity to thank my family for their support and encouragement in my decision to write this book.

A special thank you to my sister Joanne, for taking the time and effort to help design my book cover, and also to those who have helped in other ways to make my very first book become a reality.

Last but not least, a massive thank you to my best friend, soul mate and boyfriend Andrew, for giving me the inspiration to get started on this journey, and for his continued support and encouragement along the way. I am always and forever grateful to have you in my life.

My love to you ALL always!
Julie

Contents

Introduction

Welcome to *WORK WITH IT: My Hair Growth Story – Simple Steps Towards Growing Healthy Afro Hair*! This book, based on my real life experiences, contains information that I have researched, discovered, tried and tested while embarking on my hair growth journey for the past 3 and a half years.

Having successfully managed to find a solution to my hair problems, I was asked on numerous occasions by family and friends how I had managed to grow my hair longer and to provide them with my hair growth regimes so that they could grow long healthy hair too. It eventually occurred to me that this information shouldn't just be shared amongst my family and friends but made widely available to other black women looking for answers to their own hair problems. With this inspirational thought and those women in mind, I set about putting together all the information I had learned, to help them achieve similar results.

This book has been written for women looking for solutions to their hair problems. Whether you feel your hair isn't growing any longer, whether you are suffering with constant hair breakage, whether you have been drawn into the many myths and misconceptions about our hair, or whether you have just decided to start taking better care of your hair and in search of information to help you maintain a healthier hair care regime, this book is for you.

It is completely different to any other hair care book I have read before and I have purposely designed it this way in the hope that I will be able to relate to each *individual* reader in one way or another. I want to share my first hand experiences with you and in doing this, I hope to provide you with a more personal approach that encourages, motivates and inspires you to get started on your hair growth journey while eliminating any self-doubt or disbelief that afro hair does not grow or cannot grow long.

Using the simple methods and techniques contained within this book, I will show you (step by step) what I did to grow long, healthier hair and how I achieved my hair growth goals way beyond what I had ever expected. Most importantly, I want you to see and read the experiences, struggles and lessons I learnt, because there will always be many hurdles in trying to achieve anything you set out to do in life.

I hope you enjoy reading my book.

Best Wishes,

Julie Oli

Chapter 1
How It All Started

I had always thought that I had long hair but as I got to the age of around 16 or 17 I began to notice that my hair never really grew more than a few inches past my neck and I often wondered why. I eventually accepted the fact that my hair would probably never grow any longer due to my genetic makeup (an explanation I had heard as being the prime reason for a person's hair length) and so my wishful thinking for long hair went sadly out the window. My hair was just about shoulder-length and, up until that point, I had never really tried anything different like having it cut short or having layers put in it. I had been too afraid to try something new in case it didn't go to plan and I'd be left with a style I'd regret. One of my older sisters had been trying various styles with her hair and it always looked good, so it gave me the confidence to try out a few things with mine and one of those things was to have it cut quite short. At the time, I didn't have as much freedom with my hair as my older sister did and my first challenge was to try and convince my mum into allowing me to cut it. I remember thinking to myself that if I could come up with a good enough reason to cut my hair then she'd let me do it. So, I told her that my hair was breaking at the back and that it would make sense to cut it shorter so that the back could catch up with the rest of my hair. She wasn't convinced and told me I couldn't. It took a long while before she eventually gave in and, I must say, I had a lot of fun trying out the various haircuts and styles throughout those years, fortunately, without any regrets.

It wasn't until one particular day I took my experimenting a bit too far and, unfortunately, experienced the worst to come. In April 2006 I decided to visit a hair salon which a friend had recommended to me. She also recommended a particular hair stylist to do my hair and I obviously trusted her judgement since she had been to this salon on many occasions and was always happy with the service she'd received. At the time I had a chin length bob, my hair was in reasonable condition and I was content with how it looked. I wasn't planning to try anything new; I just wanted to have my hair professionally done so that it would have the fresh salon look, feel, shine and movement to it.

The hair stylist washed my hair and then proceeded to blow-dry it. Once finished, she told me that my hair was a bit limp and would look good with some layers to give it some extra volume. I told her I wasn't too sure about it but she told me to trust her and that it would look good after she'd finished. I thought about it for a second thinking that some thickness to my hair would be nice as it wasn't that full in the first place but, at the same time, it had taken me a while to grow my hair to the length I had. I also wasn't sure whether I wanted to experiment anymore but despite feeling a little sceptical I decided to give it a go; after all, it couldn't be that bad and I had experimented plenty of times before.

The second the stylist began to cut into my hair I realised that I had changed my mind but it was too late. It was seeing the razor blade in her hand that threw me into turmoil because, firstly, I didn't like the fact that she was using it to cut my hair with instead of using scissors; and, secondly, it was the way she was carelessly gliding the razor blade through my hair as though she was slicing through some material for making clothes. I remember sitting in the chair and looking into the mirror watching my hair being sliced away and seeing it slowly floating from my head, down to the floor. My hair was becoming shorter and shorter by the second and being made thinner and wispy. I could feel a ball in my throat, my stomach churning with sickness while I stared into the mirror at myself with panic and distress. When she had finally finished, I ended up with this:

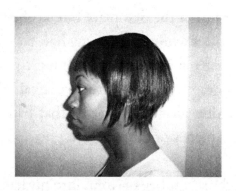

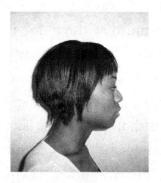
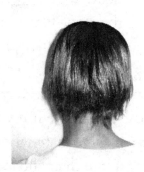

These pictures were taken a couple of weeks after the cut. I wish I had taken some before pictures so that you could see exactly how much was taken off. Based on all my bad hair salon experiences, this had to be the worst; yet, at the time when it was happening I didn't say anything. I remember the stylist bringing over the mirror at the end and holding it up so that I could look at all angles of my hair and me, like a fool, sitting there smiling and nodding my head as though I was happy with it when inside I had so many different emotions running through me. I wanted to get out of the salon as quickly as I could without anyone seeing my hair. I wanted to say to the stylist, 'What the hell have you done to my hair?' and to let her know that I wasn't happy with it, or to have refused to pay for the terrible service; but I didn't say anything because I was too embarrassed to cause a scene. After I left the salon, I was even more angry at myself as I began to think over and over again about what had just happened and how I hadn't uttered a word to let the stylist know that I hated what she had done to my hair. I couldn't understand what she was thinking to have cut my hair in that style, although it did make sense judging from the crazy hairstyle she was wearing that day. The entire sides and back of her hair were completely shaved off and she was left wearing a Mohican which shot up in the middle. I guess this should have rung alarm bells in my head from the moment I laid eyes on her.

I did learn a very good lesson that day and that was to NEVER EVER let anyone cut my hair again. I think I was even more upset when I met up with my boyfriend that very same day. The minute he saw me his face became straight and stern. I knew exactly what he was thinking moments before he opened his mouth to tell me they had 'butchered' it. My family and friends said it looked ok when they saw my hair and I thought the front of it looked fine because I liked the fringe but that was about it. The back and the sides were the problem areas for me because my hair was all different lengths. It was now much thinner than it was before and there was just no style as far as I was concerned. The cut may have been more suitable for someone looking for a funky look but it just wasn't for me and there was no hiding away from it. So I just had to put aside my upset and make good with what I had.

I found it difficult to create a variety of styles from one day to the next because there wasn't much I could do with it. I couldn't tie it in a ponytail anymore, I couldn't pin it up at the back in a French twist because it wasn't long enough, I couldn't do anything apart from wearing it the way it was. I had always wanted to grow my hair long, and I mean really long, but because of the way it was looking all I could think about was cutting it so that I could try and even out the layers to make it look more presentable and have it all grow at the same length. I then began to realise that it was never going to grow longer quickly if all I kept doing was cutting it. My main problem was that I didn't have the time or the patience to let my hair grow at its own pace; I just wanted it to happen straightaway so that I didn't have to feel the way I did about my hair and my look. My boyfriend often told me not to cut it and to let it grow because he thought longer hair would suit me, but him telling me that only annoyed me more because he didn't actually realise how much time and effort it would take to grow my hair and it wasn't going to instantly grow overnight. I ignored him and continued to do things my own way and in my own time.

Six months passed by and my hair hadn't grown much. I began thinking again about how I was going to go about growing my hair if I was really serious about doing it. At the time it just seemed like wishful thinking and longing for something that I might never be able to achieve as I couldn't realistically see how it was going to happen. Just thinking about the process of getting started was too much hassle to even contemplate, so I decided that to make things quick and easy, I was going to get a weave which would instantly give me longer hair, change my old look and allow me to give my hair a break so that it could grow. Before I knew it, I ended up wearing the weave for 10 months which wasn't supposed to be part of the plan. I had also started to notice some breakage at the front of my hair where I wore my parting to cover over the tracks and so I decided that I had to do something about it. I removed the weave and my hair hadn't grown or improved much from when I first put it in, so there wasn't much point wearing it anymore since it was causing more damage to my hair. I continued to struggle with managing my own hair while trying to figure out what my next plan of action would be.

One particular day back in August 2007, my boyfriend and I were having the usual conversation about him telling me to grow my hair, and he mentioned 3 words to me: *'Work With It'*. I thought about those words for a few seconds and it just triggered in my mind that all this time I was working against my hair rather than working with what it really wanted and needed. I decided that from that day forward I was no longer going to work against it but to *'Work With It'* and those 3 magical words changed everything for me.

I began my hair growth journey in October 2007 and this was the length I started out with:

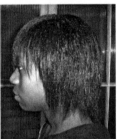

Left side view shows thinning hair at
the front and unhealthy looking hair

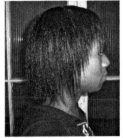

Right side view shows uneven ends
and damaged looking hair

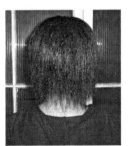

Back side view shows uneven hair
and thinning at the ends.

Chapter 2
WORK WITH IT!
The 3 Magical Words

Those 3 magical words, '*Work With It*', stuck with me from the beginning of my hair growth journey and helped me to focus on what I was going to do. The first thing I did was search the internet for as much information as I could on hair growth. I searched through various hair care forums to find out what black women were talking about on hair growth and stumbled across one called; '*Blackhairmedia.com*'. I wanted to know what other women were doing to their hair, how they were doing it and whether it was working. I saw so many women on these forums who had posted pictures of their real hair which was long, thick and right down their backs and I immediately started to doubt that it was actually their own. I made the assumption that they were wearing weaves and that it was almost impossible for some of them to even claim having the lengths I had seen. I was completely negative about it all. The majority of these women were from the USA and so I made up excuses for my ignorance telling myself things like, 'Oh...well they have softer water than we do here in the UK so that's probably why' and, 'Their hair products are better than what we have in the UK' and so on. But as I started to immerse myself deeper into the information I found, I started to find more women with nice, long hair and I began to question myself on why they would bother posting pictures if their hair wasn't real. What they would gain from doing that? There were many members on the forum posting comments to one another and congratulating each other on their hair growth achievements. Eventually, I noticed that it wasn't just women from the USA but women all over the world growing long healthy hair right down their backs. My disbeliefs about my hair not being able to grow really long slowly began to change and I started to believe that maybe it was possible to grow my hair much longer than ever before.

The next thing I searched the internet for was hair growth articles, blogs and books. There was so much information out there that I found it difficult to narrow down my choices to information that I thought would be the best sources for me. Not only did I desperately want to grow my hair longer and healthier, I was also certain from the beginning that I wasn't just going to start growing it based on the first piece of information I came into contact with. It had to be information based on what other successful hair growers were discussing and recommending to each other, and it had to be something that was definite and proven to work. So, having gathered many useful sources from the internet, I decided that it was time to purchase my first book on hair growth. This book was called, *'Ultra Black Hair Growth II by Cathy Howse'.* I had seen a fair number of women talking about her book, which made me want to find out what she had to say. I used her book as a basis for ideas and approaches that would help to add to the knowledge I had already gained from my research. With all the extensive information, I decided that it was time to put everything I had learnt into action and to create and develop a hair growth regime that would realistically work for me. I was so excited about this new venture that I couldn't wait to buy all the necessary hair tools and equipment to help me on my way.

Firstly, I made a list of all the essential facts I had learnt and believed would help me to grow my hair longer, stronger and healthier. I looked into purchasing the necessary hair tools, one being my hooded dryer; I clearly remember the day I ordered it online, eagerly awaiting its arrival. I then went about identifying the most popular hair products being used by the women on the hair forums as I was desperate to try other products that might have made my hair grow quicker. I already owned plenty of products but, in the heat of all the excitement and anticipation, I ended up buying more, almost turning my bathroom into a hair products shop!

The next step was to eliminate my old hair care habits and create completely new ones based on my new awareness. I vowed to myself that I would continue to keep growing my hair for as long as it would take me to reach my hair growth goal and never to give up no matter what.

My new hair regime consisted of the following:

- Washing my hair once a week
- Conditioning my hair after every wash
- Applying leave-in conditioners after conditioning my hair
- Air-drying my hair

- Taking hair vitamin tablets on a daily basis
- Keeping my hair moisturised as often as possible
- Carrying out the 'baggying' method
- Massaging my scalp
- Low manipulation and treating my hair with extra care
- Not greasing my scalp
- Not using hair moisturising products containing Mineral Oil/Petroleum or Short Chain Alcohols
- Limiting the use of flat irons
- Trimming my hair 1-2 times a year
- Relaxing my hair every 2 months

Implementing these new habits meant eliminating and wiping my memory of what I had been taught all my life about my hair and starting afresh, as though I was learning to manage my hair for the very first time. It was quite strange at first but exciting at the same time.

I am now going to break down each of my hair regime steps, one by one, clearly explaining why I have chosen to follow these particular methods, and the benefits they have on Afro hair.

Washing my hair once a week

Washing your hair once a week helps to remove product build up that has accumulated on the scalp from all the products that have been applied in the week. This allows new hair growth to freely grow through your scalp without anything clogging it and prevents the hair strands from feeling weighed down, clammy and lifeless. With regular washes, your hair is always left fresh, clean and generally in a healthier condition.

Conditioning my hair after every wash

There are two different methods that should be used when conditioning the hair. One is using a protein conditioner and the other is a moisturising conditioner. I ensure that I alternate between both conditioners on a weekly basis.

When carrying out a deep protein condition, I sit under my hooded dryer for 20mins. Using heat causes the hair cuticles (the outer layer of the hair) to swell open, allowing the conditioning agents to penetrate and rebuild the hair strands, making it stronger, softer and more manageable.

When carrying out a moisturising condition I simply wrap my hair in cling film and let it sit on my hair for 15-20mins. This helps to add moisture, smoothness and shine.

I talk more about protein and moisture conditioning in Chapter 3.

Applying leave-in conditioners after conditioning my hair

I use two different leave-in conditioners on my hair after washing out the conditioner. One is a protein leave-in conditioner which adds protein to my hair for strength, emollients for shine and humectants for softness; the other is a moisturising leave-in conditioner, used for detangling, protecting and naturally conditioning my hair.

I sometimes use the moisture leave-in conditioner in between hair washes, although this is not necessary.

Air-drying my hair

I prefer to air-dry my hair as often as possible to protect it from heat damage, thinning, dryness and breakage.

Regular use of a blow dryer can have harmful effects and cause breakage due to the intense heat it uses. It also removes moisture from our already dry textured hair.

Therefore, I only choose to blow dry my hair <u>twice every 2 months</u>.

Taking hair vitamin tablets on a daily basis

I take two types of hair vitamin tablets on a daily basis: Zinc and Biotin.

Zinc encourages cell division and growth. It helps to support a healthy immune system and it's also a good source of antioxidants. Biotin helps to maintain healthy skin and hair, as well as support the functioning of the nervous system. It is also known to increase the diameter of the hair strand.

There are many other vitamin tablets that can be used to aid in hair growth; however, I choose to use this combination.

Keeping my hair moisturised as often as possible

I moisturise my hair twice a day; once in the morning and once in the evening, just before I go to bed. It is very important to ensure that your hair is highly moisturised to avoid it from becoming too dry and brittle.

If you are someone who suffers from extremely dry hair and cannot appear to find a product that fully moisturises it, then you might want to check your porosity levels (see Chapter 3).

The 'baggying' method

'Baggying' is a method I discovered on the *'Blackhairmedia. com'* forum. It consists of tying your hair into a pony tail, moisturising the ends and then wrapping it in cling film or a small plastic food bag and leaving it on overnight. This helps to keep the ends of your hair highly moisturised and is important in helping to retain length.

You must remember, if the ends of your hair are always dry it will eventually lead to breakage and you will forever be trying to gain length.

MOISTURE IS KEY!

Massaging my scalp

Massaging your scalp is a good way of getting blood to flow to the hair follicles. The massaging process stimulates the hair cells which, in turn, deliver nutrients to the hair follicles to assist with hair growth.

I like to massage my scalp using various different oils which I refer to in Chapter 10.

Low manipulation and treating my hair with extra care

I am always very gentle when combing my hair, especially now that it has become a lot longer. I also avoid unnecessary combing and manipulating. I comb my hair from the ends, up towards the root, as opposed to from the root down to the ends. It is necessary to do this in order to free up the hairs as you work your way up, making it more manageable and minimising breakage.

Combing your hair from the root down with force can rip out or snap your hair because the strands get caught and tangled on themselves very easily. Afro hair is already quite delicate and naturally dry so it doesn't take much for this to happen. Always comb with extra care.

One quick tip: Now this might not suit everyone but since I'm sharing all my tips with you I may as well tell you this one too. I only <u>fully</u> comb my hair from the <u>root</u> on hair wash days, and for the rest of the week I just slightly comb and brush up the sides and back. Doing this prevents my hair from undergoing the everyday stresses and strains that combing and styling has on our hair and, in many cases, can cause breakage if not conducted in the right way.

"The less you manipulate your hair, the more you will keep on your head."

Not greasing my scalp

Hair grease actually clogs and blocks up the pores in the scalp, causing a stunt in hair growth and has no real benefit to the hair. Our scalp naturally produces its own oil, known as sebum, which prevents hair from drying out. However, due to our very tight afro curl pattern these oils have great difficulty in fully nourishing the entire hair strands (from root to tip) which leaves us with the driest hair type of all races.

Our hair actually needs moisture and <u>not grease.</u>

Not using hair moisturising products containing Mineral Oil/Petroleum or Short Chain Alcohols.

I do not use any hair moisturising products containing mineral oil (also known as petroleum) or short chain alcohols for the following reasons:

Mineral oil contains both moisture and oil, with oil being the most overpowering ingredient of the two. When combined together, mineral oil simply coats the hair preventing moisture from getting in, leaving your hair dry.

There are many different types of alcohols contained in hair products. Some are known as 'short chain alcohols', (which are bad for your hair), and others known as long chain, or fatty alcohols, (which are good for your hair).

Short Chain Alcohols are used as a preservative to maintain longer shelf life of a product. They are also used to help decrease the amount of time it takes for hair to dry. The bad thing about them is they remove moisture from the hair which causes the hair cuticles to roughen, leaving it prone to dryness.

The moisturising products I use contain *cetearyl alcohol* which is a long chain alcohol and helps to hydrate the hair rather than dry it out.

Limited use of flat-irons

I limit my usage of flat-irons to <u>once every 2 months.</u> Flat-ironing your hair often can cause breakage due to high heat, especially if you are flat-ironing on hair that is not clean or is extremely dry and brittle.

To minimise breakage or damage, it is important that you flat-iron on clean hair, use a heat protectant, use low to medium heat settings and ensure your hair is moisturised during the whole process.

Trimming my hair

Trimming your hair often to make it grow thicker and faster is a theory I've been used to hearing most of my life and has never worked for me. One thing it has done is to prevent me from gaining longer hair lengths.

I only trim my hair <u>once or twice a year</u> and ensure that I keep up with my hair care regime. I retain more length in trimming it once a year, than I have done when I used to trim it regularly.

I talk more about 'trimming hair' in Chapter 7

Relax my hair every 2 months

I used to relax my hair every 6 weeks but now I do it every 2 months. The reason for this is to allow my hair enough time to recuperate from the harsh chemical content and allow extra time in between relaxers which cause instant damage to our hair.

If possible, stretch your relaxers to 2 months or more, but remember stretching for too long can sometimes cause breakage. Therefore, it is important to know how much your hair can tolerate before it gets to this point.

To show you how effective my above methods are here is a picture of my hair length at the time of taking this photo in June 2011:

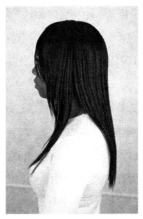

Left side view shows fuller hair at the
front and much longer and healthier.

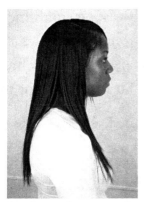

Right side view shows even ends and
no longer damaged looking hair.

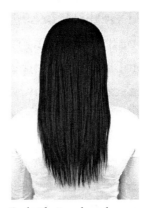

Back side view shows longer,
stronger, healthy hair.

When I compare these pictures to my starting out length in October 2007, it truly amazes me how far I have come, and I'm grateful that I was able to achieve a goal which appeared to be an impossible one back then.

All these methods have been vital to my hair growth success and if I chose to eliminate a few of them on the list I believe it would have affected my hair growth results. To be able to achieve similar results your mentality can not be one that thinks, 'Ok, I'm going to wash and condition my hair this week and leave it for another 2-3 weeks before I wash it again' or 'I'm going to apply some of the methods but I don't need to apply them all'. The reason why I say this is because you'll be wasting your time and will be forever trying to grow your hair longer. It's about a combination of processes that make a greater impact when used consistently together. So, if you're going to do this then do it whole heartedly.

To get you started on your own hair growth journey, in Chapter 3, I have outlined my hair growth regimes for you to easily duplicate.

Chapter 3
My Easy Peasy Hair Growth System

O k, so you want to grow your hair and you're looking for the easiest way to get you started? Well that's great because I have made things simple by enclosing <u>two</u> of my many different hair growth regimes for you to follow. Using these proven hair methods which I still use today, I will help get you started on your own hair growth journey with confidence and ease.

Please note: I have disclosed the hair products I use on my hair <u>as a guide only</u>, so please feel free to use your own products during this activity.

My hair regimes consist of:

- Weekly hair treatments
- Relaxer days
- Daily hair care
- Nightly hair care

The most important thing is that you stick to these regimes until you start noticing some results and have enough knowledge and confidence to make some small changes of your own.

Please note: I have purposely repeated several important hair processes for you to remember what you must do.

So, let's get started!

Wash Week 1 – Protein Treatment

- Wet your hair under the shower until your whole head is wet.

- Apply *VO5 Deep Nourishing Elixir with Cashmere Keratin Strengthening Shampoo* to your hair and massage your entire head, concentrating on the scalp. You can also apply a very small amount to the ends of your hair but your focus point is washing your scalp, not the ends. Do not use your nails to scratch your scalp, just use your fingertips. Only shampoo once.

- Rinse out the shampoo completely and squeeze out the excess water with your hands.

- Use your towel and pat your hair to dry it - <u>DO NOT rigorously rub the towel over your hair</u> as this can cause breakage because hair is very fragile when wet.

- Apply *Organics Olive Oil Replenishing Conditioner* to your hair and massage it into your scalp, ensuring that you cover your entire hair and ends. Then pin your hair up using a bobby pin and wrap your whole head in cling film or a shower cap. Sit under a hooded dryer for 20mins on high heat.

  Please note: I have a mini hooded dryer with only 2 settings so I choose the highest setting. It is good to use high heat for conditioning but select a temperature that is most comfortable for you.

- Rinse out the conditioner completely and squeeze out the excess water with your hands.

- Use your towel and <u>pat your hair to dry it - DO NOT rigorously rub the towel over your hair</u> as this can cause breakage because hair is very fragile when wet.

- Apply a combination of *Aphogee Provitamin Leave-in Conditioner* and *Aussie Miracle Hair Insurance Leave-in Conditioner* all over your hair. Ensure you cover your hair line, back of head, sides, middle sections and most importantly the ends.

- Part your hair into four sections. Comb each section from the ends up towards the root, detangling any knots. Do not pull or force the comb through your hair, be gentle.

- Pour a generous amount of *Fantasia IC Organic Tropic Fruit Anti-frizz Serum* **or** *Fantasia Hair Polisher Organic Shea Butter Moisturizing Serum* **with** *Organics Shea Butter & Tea Tree Oil Moisturiser* into the palm of your hands and rub together. Apply the mix to each sections of your hair, ensuring that you concentrate on the ends. Once all sections have been done let all sections loose.

- Allow your hair to air-dry and continue to feel it every so often. As it begins to dry, your hair will naturally soak up the moisture you have applied so you may need to apply more. I tend to use *World of Curls Comb-Out Conditioner & Oil Sheen Moisturiser* because it is really good for keeping my hair moisturised all day.

- Once your hair has dried, if necessary, apply more moisture to your hair and then tie it into a ponytail ensuring the ponytail has been fully moisturised. Next, wrap your ponytail in cling film or a small plastic food bag and leave on overnight. This helps to keep the ends moisturised preventing them from becoming dry and prone to breakage.

  (If you cannot tie your hair into a ponytail, just add enough moisture to the ends of your hair).

- Using a silk satin head scarf, fold it into a triangular shape and then place it over your head. Ensure the ends can be tied together at the back. Do not tie it too tight.

Quick tip: If your ends are continuously dry it will eventually lead to breakage. If your ends are highly moisturised they will not break. This will help you to retain length and that's when you will start noticing your hair growing longer.

Wash Week 2 – Moisturising Treatment

- Wet your hair under the shower so that your whole head is wet.

- Apply *Pantene Pro V Clarifying Shampoo* to your hair and massage your entire head concentrating on the scalp. You can also apply a very small amount to the ends of your hair but your focus point is washing your scalp. Do not use your nails to scratch your scalp, just use your fingertips. <u>Only shampoo once.</u>

Please note: Only use this shampoo once a month, as it is a clarifying shampoo which shouldn't be used often due to its harsh ingredients. It is very good for removing all traces of dirt from the scalp and helps the hair to come out squeaky clean.

- Rinse out the shampoo completely and squeeze out the excess water.

- Use your towel and pat your hair to dry it - <u>DO NOT rigorously rub the towel over your hair</u> as this can cause breakage because hair is very fragile when wet.

- Apply *Motions Moisture Plus After-shampoo Conditioner* to your hair ensuring that it covers your entire head and ends. Then pin your hair up using a bobby pin and wrap it in cling film or a shower cap and leave it on for 15-20mins. There is no need to go under the dryer. Always read the instructions on the packaging.

- Rinse out the conditioner completely and squeeze out the excess water.

- Use your towel and pat your hair to dry it - <u>DO NOT rigorously rub the towel over your hair</u> as this can cause breakage because hair is very fragile when wet.

- Apply a combination of *Aphogee Provitamin Leave-in Conditioner* **with** *Aussie Miracle Hair Insurance Leave-in Conditioner* all over your hair. Ensure you cover your hair line, back of head, sides, middle sections and most importantly the ends.

- Part your hair into four sections. Comb each section from the ends up towards the root, detangling any knots. Do not pull or force the comb through your hair, be gentle.

- Pour a generous amount of *Fantasia IC Organic Tropic Fruit Anti-frizz Serum* **or** *Fantasia Hair Polisher Organic Shea Butter Moisturizing Serum* **with** *Organics Shea Butter & Tea Tree Oil Moisturiser* into the palm of your hands and rub together. Apply the mix to each sections of your hair, ensuring that you concentrate on the ends. Once all sections have been done let all sections loose.

- Allow your hair to air-dry and continue to feel your hair every so often. As it begins to dry, your hair will naturally soak up the moisture so you may need to apply more. Be sure to repeat the above instruction if necessary.

- Once your hair has dried, if necessary, apply more moisture and then tie your hair into a ponytail ensuring the ponytail is slightly moist. Next, wrap the ponytail in cling film or a small plastic food bag and leave on overnight. This helps to keep the ends moisturised preventing them from becoming dry and prone to breakage.

- Using a silk satin head scarf, fold it into a triangular shape and then place it over your head. Ensure the ends can be tied together at the back. Do not tie it too tight.

(Make sure you alternate your weekly treatments between protein and moisture as shown above).

If you feel like trying something different with your hair like I sometimes do, rather than leaving your hair to fully dry, part it into small sections and then braid your hair. Leave it in overnight. The next morning, take out the braids and use your fingers to slowly separate the hair until all sections are evenly separated.

You will end up with little wavy curls which look like this:

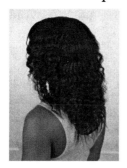 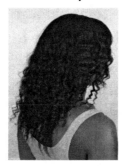 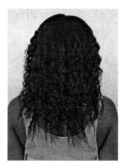

Please note: Only conduct your treatments using heat when the label on the packaging instructs you to do so. I once used heat when I wasn't supposed to and my hair felt hard, dry, was very tangled and difficult to comb.

Next, I have outlined everything I do on a daily and nightly basis for my hair care regime.

Daily hair care

- Apply a generous amount of moisturising cream to your hair concentrating on the front, back, sides and ends of hair. Be sure to apply enough moisture to last throughout the day.

- Gently comb your hair from the ends up towards the root using a large tooth comb. Ensure you are not forcing the comb through your hair, to avoid any tangles and unnecessary hair breakage.

- Create your desired style and finish.

Nightly hair care

- Using any oil of your choice, gently massage your scalp using your fingertips rotating towards the front, back, sides and middle sections of your hair. Do this for 2-5mins.

- Apply a generous amount of moisturising cream to your hair concentrating on the front, back, sides and ends of your hair. <u>Don't forget the middle sections.</u>

- Tie your hair into a ponytail ensuring the ends are slightly moist. Next, wrap the ponytail in cling film or a small plastic food bag and leave on overnight. Again, if you have short hair, just ensure the ends are moist.

- Using a silk satin head scarf, fold it into a triangular shape and then place it over your head. Ensure the ends can be tied together at the back. Do not tie it too tight.

Relaxer days

Relaxer days are slightly different to normal wash days since harmful chemicals are being applied to my hair. I relax my hair with *Organic Root Stimulator Olive Oil Built-in Protection 'No lye' Relaxer* and I buy *regular strength* since my scalp is very sensitive. This relaxer comes in a package with shampoo, wrap set mousse and a moisturiser.

Before I relax my hair, there are <u>two</u> important processes I always ensure I carry out prior to the relaxer treatment:

Deep protein treatment

A week before a relaxer is due I carry out a deep protein treatment. I do this to rebuild and strengthen my hair strands so that they are strong enough to endure and withstand the chemicals contained in the relaxer. If, for any reason, I carry out a moisturising treatment the week before a relaxer is due then I will not relax my hair. Instead, I'll postpone it for an extra week. Protein provides our hair's strength and structure so this is a vital step in the process of preventing breakage. If your hair is weak or damaged prior to the relaxing process and is not correctly maintained afterwards it will eventually lead to more breakage.

Basing hair with oils

I always base or apply oils to my hair before relaxing it to guard it against the sodium hydroxide contained within the relaxer. This chemical is responsible for breaking down the protein bonds in the hair damaging its structure and is an on-going process from the moment the relaxer is applied to the hair, up until the point when it has been completely washed out. Applying the oils, acts as a barrier between the hair and the relaxer, guarding it from fully penetrating the strands. I do not apply the oils to my scalp or roots otherwise the relaxer will not work properly.

Once my hair has been prepped and the relaxer has been applied to my regrowth, I then proceed to do the following;

- Immediately wash off and remove as much of the relaxer as possible.

- Shampoo my hair (minimum 3 times) with the Olive Oil Creamy Aloe Neutralizing Shampoo that comes with the relaxer kit.

Please note: On relaxer days it is important to shampoo (at least) 3 times to ensure that all the relaxer has been removed completely.

The next stage is as follows;

- Use your towel and pat your hair to dry it - <u>DO NOT rigorously rub the towel over your hair</u> as this could cause breakage because hair is very fragile when wet.

- Apply the *Olive Oil Replenishing Pack Conditioner* (that comes in the box) to your hair ensuring that it covers your entire head and ends. Then pin your hair up and wrap it in cling film or a shower cap. Sit under the hooded dryer for 20mins.

- Rinse out the conditioner completely and then squeeze out the excess water with your hands.

- Use your towel and *pat* your hair to dry it - <u>DO NOT rigorously rub the towel over your hair</u> as this can cause breakage because hair is very fragile when wet.

- Spray *Aphogee Keratin & Green Tea Spray* (recommended after every chemical treatment) **with** *Aussie Miracle Hair Insurance Leave-in Conditioner* all over your hair ensuring that you cover your hair line, back of head, sides, middle sections and most importantly the ends.

- Part your hair into four sections. Comb each section from the ends up towards the root, detangling any knots. Do not pull or force the comb through your hair, be gentle.

- Apply a generous amount of *Fantasia IC Organic Tropic Fruit Anti-frizz Serum* **or** *Fantasia Hair Polisher Organic Shea Butter Moisturizing Serum* (which are both good heat protectants) to each section of your hair. Proceed to blow-dry slowly on low or medium heat, starting from the ends and working your way up towards the roots.

- Once all four sections have been blow-dried, let your hair loose and re-blow-dry the areas which are still damp until all sections are completely dry.

- Before flat ironing your hair apply more *Fantasia IC Organic Tropic Fruit Anti-frizz serum* **or** *Fantasia Hair Polisher Organic Shea Butter Moisturizing Serum* to replace lost moisture from blow-drying.

- Starting from the back, part your hair into small sections and flat-iron. Then style as normal.

Please note: I only run the flat-iron over my hair once.

- If necessary, you can add more *Fantasia IC Organic Tropic Fruit Anti-frizz Serum* **or** *Hair Polisher Organic Shea Butter Moisturizing Serum* **with** *some Organics Shea butter & Tea Tree Oil Moisturiser* for smoothness and shine.

If you are self-relaxing it is advisable that you follow the step by step instructions that come with the relaxer kit or have a professional do it for you.

To accurately monitor your hair growth results, take pictures of your hair at the very beginning of your hair growth journey and continue to do so every 2 months. This way you get to measure the growth you have achieved during those months. It's a great idea to do this because it will give you great motivation to continue going, especially when you start noticing results. It's only when you see the results that you become aware that your hair is actually growing and I say this because I felt the exact same way when I was going through the process myself.

Alternating your Protein & Moisture Treatments

It is important to have an even balance of both protein and moisture treatments. If your hair receives too much moisture it eventually becomes too elasticated causing your hair to overstretch when combed, leading to breakage. On the other hand, if you apply too much protein the opposite occurs; your hair becomes less elasticated causing it to be less resilient to stretching which means it can break very easily too. Maintaining a balance between the two treatments ensures that your hair is stable and less likely to break.

Porosity Levels

Porosity is another important factor in hair care. It determines how easily your hair can absorb and retain moisture and there are 3 levels of porosity; low, normal and high.

See diagram 1.1 below showing the 3 various stages;

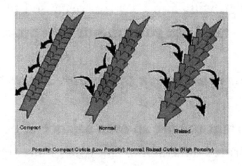

Porosity: Compact Cuticle (Low Porosity); Normal; Raised Cuticle (High Porosity)

Low porosity (also known as compact) is when your hair finds it difficult to absorb moisture due to how tightly closed your cuticle layers lay. Normal porosity is when your hair finds it easy to absorb and retain moisture; since the cuticle layer is slightly open allowing for moisture to enter in and out. High porosity (also known as raised) is when your hair is able to absorb lots of moisture but does not retain it due to how raised the cuticle layers are positioned.

So what exactly determines your hair's porosity level, you may ask? Well, it all boils down to the structure of your cuticle (the outer layer of your hair) and the processes you undertake that affect them. For example; regularly blow drying, flat ironing, colour treating and using chemical relaxers in your hair causes your cuticle layer to raise and become exposed resulting in constant moisture imbalance. To keep your hair at normal level, minimise the use of heat, colour treatments and chemical treatments on your hair and ensure the PH balance of your hair is evenly balanced between acidic and alkaline products.

PH Balance

PH stands for Potential Hydrogen and is measured on a scale of 0 – 14; 0 being most acidic and 14 being most alkaline. All hair products are measured along this scale, some falling closer to the acidic side, some neutral and others on the alkaline side of the scale. The PH balance of hair is between, 4.5 and 5.5. Knowing roughly where your hair products fall along this scale will help to ensure your hair is kept close to the correct balance.

Products that have a PH balance of around 8 and above raise the cuticle layers and anything from 4 downwards close the cuticle layers. Now, for those of us who relax or colour treat our hair the bad news is that these chemicals increase the PH balance of the hair to as high as 11-14, leaving the cuticle layers wide open resulting in moisture loss and dry hair prone to breakage. That is why it is so important to use a neutralising shampoo immediately after chemically treating your hair, to bring the PH balance back down.

Below is a diagram showing a PH scale:

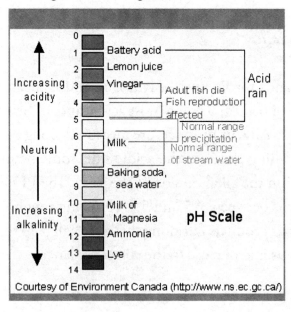

Looking at the scale you will notice that lemon juice and vinegar will help to close the cuticle layers of your hair, and Ammonia and Lye raise the cuticle layers. The hair products you use on your hair determine whether your hair will have low, normal or high porosity.

To check the correct PH balance of your hair products, you may want to purchase your own PH testing kit to accurately test each product.

Chapter 4
When Things Get Tough,
Don't Give Up!

S o, how badly do you really want to grow your hair on a scale of 1-10? Everyone wants a lot of things but how many people really have the drive, passion and determination to get there? Not many. It's all very exciting when you know something is possible because you've seen it or you personally know someone who has managed to do it. But when you really get down to the nitty gritty and the hard work, it can take many people by surprise and that's when they fall by the way side.

So you have to think about the reasons for wanting to grow your hair and make a decision from the offset to commit to doing so. For example; is it because you have a special occasion coming up and you need to reach your hair growth goal by this date? Maybe it's because you just want to achieve longer lengths so you don't have to wear weaves or braids anymore? Or is it because you actively want to start taking better care of your hair for the long term? Whatever your reasons for growing it, just make sure you're committed to the process.

Now that my hair is much longer I do notice people staring at it, trying to figure out whether or not it's my real hair. I've been approached a few times and asked whether my hair is real. One person asked me what weave I was wearing while another commented on how good the quality of my weave was. I had to let them know that it was all mine. Many people who do not know me, or who had never seen my hair when I first started out, would automatically assume that I've always had really long hair and that growing long hair has been quite easy to do. It's easy for those assumptions to be made because they're not fully aware of my story and the hard work and effort I've had to put in behind the scenes for the past 3 and a half years.

I used to work with someone who would often admire and comment on my hair saying things like, 'I'm so jealous of your hair' and 'I wish I had your hair' and I often told her that she could if she took the time to apply some effort. But she wasn't interested in finding out about how she could grow her own hair because she never asked me the *'how'* question. Maybe she didn't have the belief that it was possible for her to have long hair or maybe she just couldn't be bothered with all the hassle. I had only ever known her to wear weaves and braids so I can only guess that she had been so used to wearing these styles for so long that they had become a comfort blanket for her. Everyone has a choice and I'm not here to judge her or anyone else; the only point I would like to make is that growing your own hair long is possible; it just depends on whether you really want to and how much effort you're willing to put in to achieve the results.

As I mentioned earlier, the first year of growing my hair was the toughest because I had just embarked on my hair growth journey and knew absolutely nothing about growing my hair in the right way. What I did know was that if I was going to give this my best shot I had to drop all the old hair care habits I had been using for most of my life immediately.

Below I have made a list of my bad hair care habits. See if you can identify with any of them:

- Relaxing my hair every 6 weeks
- Washing my hair every 6 weeks
- Greasing my scalp regularly
- Blow drying my hair often
- Going to the hair salon often
- Regularly flat ironing my hair
- Combing and manipulating my hair too much
- Not moisturising my hair often enough
- Spraying my hair with Oil sheen
- Using hair gels
- Using moisturising products containing Mineral Oil/Petroleum and Short Chain Alcohols
- Cutting my hair too often
- Tying my hair too tight
- Wrapping my hair
- Using hair tights or a cotton head scarf to cover my hair at night

I'm pretty sure there were many other bad habits I had been keeping, although I cannot remember many of them now. The fact that I was able to immediately drop these habits was quite impressive, if I must say, but I think it helped that I clearly knew the reasons for wanting to grow my hair. In the back of my mind, I did wonder how long this journey was going to take and I was also doubtful about whether my hair would actually grow to the ideal length I had in my mind. I remember standing in front of the mirror one particular day, looking at my hair, thinking, 'Gosh, I've got a huge challenge ahead of me' just before my boyfriend came up from behind me asking me to try on one of his caps. He mentioned how good it would look on me once I had my long hair and I smiled because he believed it was possible, even though I wasn't as optimistic. Just hearing him say those words helped me to embody a more positive attitude and approach towards achieving my goal, and sometimes we need that moral support to keep us going.

Going back to the beginning of my hair journey I had a lot of issues with styling my hair. My most regular and worn out style having it pinning up at the back in a French twist, with a sweep fringe at the front, was worn for months and months on end, and I started to get so sick and tired of how I looked that I wondered how long I would have to endure this torture before I eventually went insane. There were days when the hairstyle looked ok and there were days when the re-growth started to show and I felt really rough and unattractive. It made me feel so insecure about myself to the point where I didn't want to look anyone in the eye. It didn't help that I was the kind of person who always had to look good whenever I was going anywhere (which wasn't necessarily a bad thing) but I had to put aside my vanity and remind myself of why I was doing it and continue to visualise how I would look once I had reached my goal. The biggest lesson I learnt from the whole experience was being comfortable with who I am as a person and not worrying so much about what people might think or have to say about me. I knew I had a goal to achieve and, despite everything else, I stuck to it.

I spoke to a friend, not so long ago, who was praising me about how well I had come along with my hair growth journey. She has regularly kept track of my hair growth progress over the years and is constantly amazed at how much my hair has grown whenever she views my latest pictures and, knowing that she admires my hair, I didn't mind her taking the opportunity to tell me some home truths about what she really thought of it way back in the early stages. She took me back to a time when we were having an evening out with the girls and she recalled how my hair had looked rough and nothing like how it normally look and she wondered what was going on with it. At the time she didn't want to ask me in case I became offended. She began to get carried away mentioning a few other comments about my hair which didn't bother me, because it was only at that point, was she able to realise, understand and appreciate how dedicated I was to achieving my goal.

I don't remember that particular time she was referring too but I'm sure I must have thought my hair was looking just fine. Either way, I do know that there have been many days when I haven't been too bothered with my hair and worn it in whatever style I felt fit. Overall, I am happy to say that I never gave up, no matter how hard it was along the way. I made a decision from the beginning about what I wanted, I focused on it and I just kept going; and that's what you have to do if you truly want to achieve something. You will encounter some struggles, possible setbacks, trials and tribulations, but that's all part of the journey. If you can find the focus and determination to push through those barriers, only then will you notice the results. You just have to be willing to invest your time, patience and effort and, believe me, it's a good feeling when you start noticing a difference.

Chapter 5
Be Lead Only By Example

I have always been a firm believer in listening to and following those who can lead by example. When I used to visit the hair salon, I always hoped that my hair would be washed and styled by the stylist with the nicest hair because I often thought, 'Well, if their hair is nice then they will know how to treat mine in order to make it grow'. But it hardly ever happened that way and I would end up having it done by someone whose hair didn't look that great. I was also given occasional advice on how to manage my hair, the most popular one being to trim it every 4-6 weeks so that it would grow. Now, how many of us have heard that saying before? And still continue to hear that today? I was also advised to have a treatment every 2 weeks to improve my hair's condition and to make it grow, but when I looked at the hair on some of the stylists who were advising me I often wondered why their real hair was never on show and instead hidden underneath weaves and braids. Surely if they knew how to maintain and care for my hair, and had been personally applying the methods they had provided me with, their own hair would be healthy, long and right down their backs, right? But it wasn't the case and this was a question that pondered in my mind. I couldn't make any sense of why someone would tell me to do something that wasn't actually working for them. In spite of that, I did sometimes take note of what I was told, mainly because I didn't know any better and I certainly wasn't aware of the information I now know today. Having applied some of the methods I was told and still seeing no results I just accepted that my hair stylists couldn't really have known the correct processes about caring for my hair and I eventually learnt to accept that the information offered was just part of the service. I remember the standard culture and services I received when I used to visit the hair salon and a number of them that were damaging to my hair.

Here are just a few of them I would like to highlight:

- Relaxers left on the hair for longer than 10mins so that it can 'take' better.
- Towels rigorously rubbed over wet, fragile hair.
- Hair blow-dried on the highest temperature and flat ironed using oven tongs.

- Hair combed from roots to ends with a small tooth comb.
- Hair wrapped 'wet' or 'dry' before going under a hooded dryer

I'll breakdown these points to let you know why I believe they are no good for your hair:

Relaxer left on the hair for longer than 10mins so that it can 'take' better

I've experienced, numerous times in the past, a relaxer being left on my hair for longer than 10 minutes to the point where I would start to feel the tingling sensation which indicated it was time to wash it off. It should never be a case of waiting to reach this stage because the sodium hydroxide in the relaxer can cause scalp burns which form into scabs or, even worst, can end up penetrating deep into the scalp causing the root to become permanently damaged, resulting in hair loss.

It can also cause over processing which leads to your hair becoming drier, weaker and more prone to breakage, especially if you do not keep up the correct hair care maintenance afterwards.

Towels rigorously rubbed over wet, fragile hair

Your hair is in its most fragile and delicate state when it is wet. Obviously, once you have finished washing your hair you must dry it using a towel. However, I find the way this is carried out extremely harsh on the hair. This is because the towel is rigorously rubbed over the hair when wet, which can easily cause the hair to snap or tear unnecessarily.

You only need to pat the towel on your hair and squeeze the ends until dry (as mentioned in Chapter 3).

Hair blow-dried on the highest temperature and flat-ironed using oven tongs

I am not a big fan of blow-drying my hair on the highest heat setting or having my hair flat-ironed using oven tongs. Regular usage of high heat, no matter the appliance, can cause your hair to become excessively dry, thin and cause split ends that eventually lead to breakage.

Try replacing your blow-drying temperatures with a low to medium heat setting, replacing the oven tongs with flat irons on a lower setting and reduce your usage of thermal appliances to once or twice a month.

Hair combed from roots to ends with a small tooth comb

Combing your hair from the roots to the ends with a small tooth comb is the worst possible way to comb your hair. Instead, your hair should be gently combed from the ends up towards the roots using a large tooth comb.

This helps to avoid any possible tangles or knots forming which can cause your hair to be pulled or ripped out. Although we naturally lose around 100 hairs a day, many people lose a lot more simply down to the way they comb their hair.

Hair wrapped 'wet' or 'dry' before going under a hooded dryer

Wrapping your hair before going under the dryer results in a nice smooth finish but it requires a lot of manipulation to the hair, with the constant combing and brushing, until your hair is finally in place. The problem with this is that our hair doesn't like to be tampered with and too much of this causes your hair to start thinning.

For those of you who choose to visit the hair salon, I'm pretty sure you will experience these processes without even realising it and if you want to start growing your hair longer, stronger and healthier then you may want to instruct or guide your stylist on how you would like your hair to be managed. Alternatively, you can decide to take care of it yourself.

Further reading on various hair growth books is also advisable until you eventually start to notice a pattern forming in the information you'll find. You will notice that a lot of the good sources will teach similar principles but be careful as you may also come across ones that teach damaging hair care practices. To make things simpler, look and listen to women who actually have long, healthy hair and do not take advice from those whose results do not reflect what they preach.

I always used to wonder why it was only black women struggling with hair growth issues, but now I've come to realise that we have been conditioned into bad hair care practices for most of our lives. Unfortunately, these habits have been passed on from generation to generation, leaving us exposed to processes that have caused continuous hair breakage and prevention from achieving longer lengths. So now you have to ask yourself these questions: 'Am I happy with the results I'm getting?' and 'Is what I'm currently doing working for me?' If not, then you must change the way you care for your hair! It makes no sense in continuing to do something that has never worked all these years, but it makes sense to try something completely new that 'works' and will change your results for the better.

I simply made the conscious decision to make a change from something that wasn't working for me, to something that I thought was worth giving a try; and, in doing so, I have been able to achieve amazing hair growth results.

Chapter 6
What Has Genetics
Got To Do With It?

Genetics does determine many aspects of our physical appearance, however, when it comes to things such as weight and hair length, I believe that we have as much control over them as we do with anything else in life. Many people struggle to grow their hair and put it down to genetics, but if they really took the time and effort to delve deeper into these issues and investigate the problems further through research, they could possibly combat many of the struggles faced in growing and maintaining healthy hair.

Here is an example I would like to share with you about two siblings. They both have the same parents, therefore, share the same genetic makeup. One suffers with on-going breakage and scalp problems and the other doesn't suffer with either of these problems.

Let's have a look at their everyday habits:

Sibling 1	Sibling 2
• Drinks alcohol on a regular basis	• Hardly drinks alcohol
• Doesn't maintain a healthy diet	• Maintains a healthy diet
• Is a regular smoker	• Doesn't smoke
• Doesn't take good care of their hair	• Takes good care of their hair
• Doesn't drink water regularly	• Drinks water regularly
• Doesn't exercise regularly	• Exercises regularly

Compare both of their habits. Can you notice any reasons why Sibling 1 might be suffering with breakage and scalp problems and Sibling 2 doesn't? I purposely used this example to make a valid point that genetics doesn't always have something to do with it. Sometimes it's more about what we might be doing to our bodies that actually affects us.

Vitamins, proteins and minerals are nutritional supplements essential for hair growth and many of the foods available to us contain these nutrients. However, due to busy lifestyles, convenience and, in many cases, bad habits, we lack many of the important ingredients in our diet which ends up having an effect on our hair growth rate and the overall condition of our hair. Remember, our bodies need the right foods to correctly function and do their job, just like plants need sufficient water to survive and grow.

So how exactly do these bad habits affect our hair growth?

Alcohol

High levels of estrogen in the body can lead to hair loss and drinking high doses of alcohol (whether over the course of a week or in one night) increases your levels of estrogen. Alcohol affects the nutrients in your hair causing it to break. It is also known to reduce the levels of zinc in the body which is a mineral helping to promote healthy hair growth.

Diet

Maintaining a healthy and balanced diet is what keeps the body functioning correctly. A diet that contains all the necessary proteins, fibres and whole grains such as; fruit & veg, fish, chicken, dairy products, nuts and cereals, will help to keep your hair healthy.

Smoking

For hair to grow at a healthy rate it must receive the right amount of nutrients and minerals to the hair cells. Smoking affects the supply of blood circulating throughout the body and restricts vital nutrients from being delivered to the hair cells, preventing hair growth.

Hair maintenance

Keeping up with a consistent hair care regime is important for long term hair health and growth. Washing and conditioning your hair on a regular basis, alternating your moisture and protein treatments, keeping your hair highly moisturised and following the detailed hair care regimes outlined in this book will help provide long term benefits to your hair.

Drinking water

Drinking water regularly is good for your health because it helps to keep the blood circulating around the body. Water keeps the body hydrated and aids the blood in carrying oxygen and nutrients to other body cells.

Exercise

Exercise is another good way of increasing blood flow to the scalp which, again, helps to assist nutrients in reaching the hair cells in order to stimulate hair growth. A really good workout will help you to sweat, allowing your body to release toxins which act as a cleansing treatment for the scalp.

Regular exercise also helps to reduce cortisone, a hormone in the body that presents itself when you become stressed and can cause your hair to become thin or fall out.

Overall, it is very important to incorporate holistic health practices alongside your healthy hair care regime because everything we do has a great impact on our bodies. Becoming consciously aware of these habits will help you to make better lifestyle choices.

I have read many articles and blogs in the past that have spoken about how our hair will stop at a certain length due to our genetic makeup and that it can never grow past the length that has been genetically set. But, if you stop and think about that for a minute, you should be asking yourself, 'How can I know how long my hair will genetically grow if I've never known how to grow it to actually test that theory?' There are so many people out there thinking that they have reached their peak length when they haven't really given themselves the opportunity to find out. I know that if I had accepted this to be the case then I wouldn't have embarked on my hair growth journey and would never have known that my hair could grow as long as it is today.

Myths like this encourage people to have limiting beliefs about having long hair and so they give up and accept what they hear when there is no evidence to prove it. That's why I say that it is so important to educate yourself further.

Chapter 7
The Common Myths

There are so many myths that surround Afro hair which have affected us a great deal and had a huge impact on our everyday hair care habits. These myths have been embedded into our subconscious from as early as we can remember and although many of them have no real meaning or purpose, you won't realise it until you become aware of the truth.

Now, if you are not aware of these myths then you can easily be fooled into believing them. You will continue to follow these bad hair care habits, like a hamster on a wheel, going through the cycle of hair growth, hair breakage, hair growth, hair breakage, over and over again.

I have made a list of the common myths that I remember hearing when I was growing up. I have also asked some family members and friends in order to capture some of the most popular myths to get an overall view of the false information out there surrounding Afro hair.

So let's have a look at them:

- Afro hair doesn't grow and can't grow past a certain length.
- You should trim your hair every 4-6 weeks to make it grow thicker and faster.
- If you don't trim your hair often it leads to split ends that will split all the way to your hair shaft and break off.
- Washing your hair too often will dry it out and cause it to break.
- Applying grease to the scalp is good for your hair.
- If you go swimming often your hair will break.
- Braiding your hair will make it grow.
- You should relax your hair every 4-6 weeks.

Well, ladies, I can tell you that the above are all simply MYTHS and I'll explain why based on my own tried, tested and proven methods.

Afro hair doesn't grow and can't grow past a certain length

If you are alive right now, then your hair is growing and it's as simple as that. Those of you who relax your hair, think about why you do it? Ok, you want it to be straighter and more manageable, but why do you continue to relax it every 6 weeks, 2 months, 6 months or however long you decide to wait between relaxers? Because of new-growth, which means your hair is growing.

Now the reason it may appear not to grow past a certain length is down to how well you maintain your hair, as well as how often you cut it. Cutting your hair too often limits it growing potential.

You should trim your hair every 4-6 weeks to make it grow faster and thicker

This is not true; and in the first year of growing my hair I didn't trim my hair once. Why? Because I wanted to see the full length and growth that I could achieve without any restrictions, and I can confirm that it didn't do any harm to my hair; it just showed me that my hair did grow. Also, hair grows from the root and not from the ends so how trimming can possibly make it grow thicker and faster is something I will never understand.

It's a fact that the average person's hair grows at a rate of half an inch a month; in a year that's 6 inches.

So, let's say for example; that you decide to trim off half an inch of hair every month. That half an inch that you trim off sets you back by a month of possible hair growth. Then the next month comes around and you've grown another half an inch of hair and you decide to trim that half an inch off too and you continue to repeat that same pattern over and over again. What do you think is happening to your hair growth cycle? Well, NOTHING! Because every time your hair grows you cut it off which means your hair length can only stay the same as you started with. You shouldn't really be surprised why it appears not to be growing because you're not allowing the growth cycle to continue. Now, remember that's just an example. In the real world, most people I know that have their hair trimmed at the hair salon end up having 1 or 2 inches cut off. I'll leave you to work out how much that sets you back. But put it this way, at that rate, how on earth are you ever going to grow your hair down your back?

I bumped into a friend of mine, about a year ago, who I'd always known to have nice, long, healthy looking hair. When I saw her, the first thing I noticed was her hair looking a lot shorter so I assumed she had cut it. When I spoke to her I said, 'Oh, you cut your hair?' and she said, 'No, I got it trimmed at the hair salon but they ended up cutting off too much.' I asked, 'Well why did you let them do that?' She shrugged her shoulders and reluctantly said, 'Well, it's only hair' but I could clearly see that she wasn't happy about it. I knew how she was feeling because I'd experienced worse. I had never felt like I was in control of how my hair was managed when I used to visit the hair salon and I tended to go along with how the stylist was used to managing my hair, even if I didn't like the experience. I didn't want to come across as being a difficult or fussy customer so chose to sit quietly. Due to many of these uncomfortable experiences I eventually stopped going altogether and have been taking care of my hair myself.

If you don't trim your hair often it leads to split ends that will split all the way to your hair shaft and break off

When it comes to split ends you firstly need to know what causes the problem in order to minimise it. Split ends are due to many everyday processes such as blow drying, flat ironing, back combing, brushing and other processes that cause stress and strain to your hair. I do not perform these processes very often and I take great care of my hair. If you are able to do the same, it will not be necessary for you to trim your hair every 4-6 weeks.

As for your hair splitting all the way to your hair shaft, this is not true. I have been growing my hair for over 3 and a half years. During this time I have probably only trimmed it 4 or 5 times and my hair is still longer, stronger and healthier than it's ever been in all my life, and it has never split all the way to my hair shaft.

Washing your hair too often will dry it out and cause it to break

This is not true. Our hair needs regular moisture and washing is one of the best ways to moisturise the hair, as well as drinking lots of water and using hair moisturisers. It all comes down to how well you care for your hair after you wash it.

Just to make it clear, there is a big difference between breakage and shedding. Breakage is when you have small little broken bits of hair that have broken away and shedding is when you have longer hairs that have a small bulb on the end which shows that it has come from the root of your hair.

Shedding is normal, but breakage is not good.

Applying grease to the scalp is good for your hair

Grease isn't good for the scalp because it blocks the hair follicles and doesn't allow your scalp to breath, causing a stunt in hair growth. Your scalp needs be kept clean and free from product build up so that your hair can easily grow through it.

I don't apply anything to my scalp unless I'm doing a scalp massage and I only use hair oils.

If you go swimming often your hair will break

When I was learning to swim at school we had to go swimming every week. I was too young to know about hair care and never washed the chlorine out of my hair properly and so it often broke around my hairline and at the back of my head.

What I didn't realise at the time was that when you get into a swimming pool with dry hair, your hair automatically soaks up the water (which contains chlorine) because it's moisture. But if you get into a pool with hair that is already wet and contains conditioner, the conditioner will act as a barrier to block out the chlorine from fully penetrating the hair causing breakage.

To avoid hair breakage I always shampoo my hair prior to swimming and rinse out before applying a deep conditioner. After swimming I rinse out the conditioner, re-shampoo my hair to remove the conditioner and any possible traces of chlorine and then follow up with a good protein or moisturising treatment.

Braiding your hair will make it grow

Braiding your hair doesn't necessarily make it grow since hair grows anyway, but it can be good if you want to give it a break from everyday maintenance.

The only down fall in wearing braids too often means your hair doesn't receive regular maintenance, so when it comes to removing it you will find that your hair is weaker, drier and more prone to breakage.

You should relax your hair every 4-6 weeks

It is not necessary to relax your hair every 4-6 weeks regardless of the length, but we choose how often we do it to suit our own individual needs in terms of manageability and style.

It's a good idea to try and stretch your relaxers to at least 2 months or longer to avoid over-processed, weak, dry and damaged hair.

Chapter 8
Beware Of The Ingredients You Use On Your Hair!

There are many different hair products on the market that contain harmful ingredients that are not only bad for our hair, but also for our health, and because many of us are not aware of this we innocently use them being none the wiser.

Based on my personal research, I have listed below a few ingredients to be aware of:

Mineral Oil/Petroleum

Mineral oil is difficult to absorb, clogs the pores and restricts the skin's ability to remove toxins in the body. If absorbed, the liver will break it down and pass it through the bowels where it will eventually absorb all of the fat-soluble vitamins, stealing essential compounds from the body which are non-replaceable. This could eventually lead to nutritional deficiencies.

Isopropyl Alcohol

This ingredient is commonly used for medical, pharmaceutical and cleaning purposes. It can easily be absorbed through the skin leading to harmful systemic effects. It is highly flammable in the presence of high heat or an open flame and can be found in hair dyes and colour rinse products.

Polyethylene Glycol (PEG) / Propylene Glycol (PG)

These ingredients are designed to help retain moisture in the hair. Regular usage can lead to the deterioration of protein within the cellular structure of hair. They are also known ingredients in anti-freeze, floor wax, brake and hydraulic fluid and many other products that have also been linked to many severe health problems.

Sodium Lauryl Sulfate (SLS)/ Sodium Laureth Sulfate (SLES)

These ingredients are used in shampoos and hair conditioners. The strong detergent content can cause scalp irritation, hair loss and can also strip the hair of its natural moisture. These ingredients are easily absorbed into the skin and can penetrate the heart, lungs, liver and brain.

Diethanolamine (DEA), Momoethnanolamine (MEA), Triethanolamine (TEA)

These ingredients contain a neutralizing compound (such as Cocamide DEA or Lauramide DEA) that is used to thicken shampoos to create lather. Regular and persistent usage is known to irritate and absorb itself into the skin which can lead to cancer of the liver and kidneys.

It can be very difficult to have to suddenly stop using a particular product that you have been using for so long, especially if you haven't experienced any problems with it. However, it is important to be aware of the ingredients contained within your products for your own health, safety and wellbeing even if you decide to continue using them.

Many people try to find alternative solutions to avoid these harsh ingredients making direct contact with their hair. For example; saturating ones hair in oils and leaving it in overnight prior to shampooing (also known as pre-pooing). This acts as a protective barrier against the harmful ingredients contained within the shampoo penetrating, stripping and robbing the hair of its natural oils. Some people will also use conditioners instead of shampoos when washing their hair (known as co washing) because conditioners are less harsh. Others will concoct their own hair remedies which may consist of natural ingredients like, coconut oil, shea butter, aloe vera, honey, avocadoes, lemon juice and various others. It's important to know the benefits of these products before applying them to your hair and the people who do this are fully aware of what they are doing.

Remember, everyone's hair type is different, so what might work for one person may not necessarily work for another.

Chapter 9
My Top 20 Tips To Retaining Longer Hair

So here are my top 20 tips that will help you to retain longer hair. Remember, the less breakage you experience the longer lengths you retain. There are lots of tips and each one is vital to your hair growth success.

1. Wash your hair weekly and follow up with a good treatment.

2. Ensure you alternate between protein and moisturising treatments weekly.

3. Stretch your relaxers to 2 months or more and do not leave relaxers on your hair. Always rinse off immediately.

4. When towel drying, always pat the towel on your hair, never rub rigorously.

5. Try to allow your hair to air-dry as often as possible and limit your usage of blow dryers and flat irons.

6. Always moisturise your hair twice a day and pay attention to the ends.

7. Avoid applying hair grease to your scalp.

8. Use the 'baggying method' to keep the ends of your hair moisturised.

9. Trim your hair less often.

10. Take hair vitamin tablets.

11. Eat healthily, exercise as often as possible and drink plenty of water.

12. Always comb your hair from the ends up towards the root. Never force the comb downwards through your hair.

13. Avoid unnecessary manipulation to your hair.

14. Wear protective hairstyles as often as possible.

15. Cover your hair every night using a satin silk head scarf to protect it from rigorous friction against the pillow.

16. Massage your hair for at least 2-5mins every night.

17. Avoid using moisturising hair products which contain mineral oil/petroleum or short chain alcohols.

18. Avoid using elastic bands, tight hair bands, tiny tooth combs, harsh hair brushes or sharp hair accessories that will get caught in your hair or cause tension or breakage.

19. Protect your hair from rubbing against coat collars, scarfs, back of seats, rough clothing or anything that will cause friction and breakage.

20. Treat your hair like silk and give it respect.

Chapter 10
Products I Use On My Hair

Below, I have listed the products that I use on my hair. Whether you decide to use the same ones or not is entirely your choice. I am often asked by people which products I use on my hair and I would like to say this:

"It's not the hair product that grows your hair but rather how you apply the product that makes the biggest difference!"

Any product that suits your hair needs will naturally provide you with results. Try different products and find out what works for your hair.

Shampoos

- V05 Deep Nourishing Elixir with Cashmere Keratin Strengthening Shampoo for Dry and Damaged Hair
- Aphogee Shampoo for Damaged Hair
- Pantene Pro V Clarifying Shampoo

Protein Conditioners

- Organic Olive Oil Replenishing Conditioner
- Organic Root Stimulator Hair Mayonnaise – Treatment for Damaged Hair

Moisturising Conditioners

- Motions Moisture Plus After-shampoo Conditioner
- Superdrug Coconut & Sweet Almond Intensive Conditioner
- Herbal Essence Hello Hydration Moisture & Shine Conditioner
- Aphogee Balancing Moisturiser

Protein Leave-in conditioners

- Aphogee Provitamin Leave-in Conditioner
- Aphogee Keratin & Green Tea Reconstructizer

Moisturising Leave-In Conditioners

- Aussie Luscious Long Leave-in Conditioner
- Elasta QP Leave-in H2

Moisturisers

- World of Curls Comb-Out Conditioner & Oil Sheen Moisturiser
- Organics Shea Butter & Tea Tree Oil Moisturiser
- Crème of Nature Daily Breakage Relief

Oils

- Claudie's Hair Revitalizer Gro Elixir
- Hollywood Beauty Castor Oil Hair Treatment with Mink Oil
- Organics Olive & Clove Oil Therapy
- Pure Coconut Oil
- Peppermint Oil
- Hair Growth Booster with Pro Vitamin-B5

Serum / Hair Polish

- Fantasia IC Organic Tropic Fruit Anti-Frizz Serum
- Fantasia IC Hair Polisher Organic Shea Butter Moisturizing Serum
- Organics Tea Tree Shine Strengthening Hair Polish

Many products on the market today promise instant hair growth or longer hair within a short period of time and many of us fail to realise that it's just never going to happen. Years ago I used to purchase products, solely based on the information contained on the box if it promised instant and longer hair growth. But I only ended up disappointed that it hadn't worked. I've come to realise that no product is ever going to provide results, no matter what it states or how much it costs, if you are not using it correctly.

For a long time, I had been so used to buying my hair products from my local black hair shop and would never go anywhere else to buy them. Even when I used to do food shopping at my local supermarket, I used to walk passed the hair care isles with products designed for European hair and wouldn't even bat an eyelid at the products on the shelf because I used to think they were not designed for my hair type. I now buy a number of products from those very same aisles which work well with my hair.

One thing you have to remember is that, no matter your race, hair is hair and it's all made up of the same thing. The only difference is in our texture.

Chapter 11
So, What Should I Do Now?

Ok, so you've reached the final chapter of the book and you may be feeling overwhelmed with all the information you've just read. Your next thought might be, '*So, what should I do now?*'

So, to help you, I've compiled a checklist below of what you should do to get things in order:

☐ Re-read this book and refer to it as often as necessary so that you fully understand the information contained within it.

☐ Read further books on hair growth and research relevant articles, blogs and even sign up to hair forums – (Refer to the Further Reading section).

☐ Make notes on the main points you feel will be beneficial for you to achieve your hair growth goals.

☐ Set yourself realistic hair targets and goals.

☐ Take pictures of your current hair length before you start your hair growth journey. Take pictures of the front, back and sides of your hair and keep a record of your pictures. This will help you to document your progress and achievements along the way so that you can see that your hair is growing. Continue to do this every 2 months.

☐ Make sure you have some support to keep you on track. Maybe you can work closely with a friend, relative or partner who will support you.

☐ Buy all the necessary hair tools and equipment that you need to get started.

You are now ready to begin your healthy hair care journey!

GOOD LUCK!

Conclusion

I hope that you have enjoyed reading my book which I have designed to help give you a head start on your hair growth journey. I know that when I first started mine I was hoping to find information that offered a step by step guide that was guaranteed to work and saved me time. It wasn't the case and this was the reason I incorporated Chapter 3, to save you the time, effort and worry about getting started.

The information in Chapter 3 are tried, tested and proven methods that I use on my own hair and, if you follow them as I have stated, you will eventually begin to notice a difference in your hair. I'm not saying that this is the only way you can grow your hair, because there are many different ways to achieve longer hair, but these are <u>some</u> of the methods I have used all these years and it has done wonders for me.

You should start noticing results within 2-4 months and, once you begin to master what you are doing, it's totally up to you if you wish to alter the regime to something that might work better for you. So there is nothing stopping you now from starting your own hair growth journey.

In looking back on my experiences, I now realise that everything happened for a reason and that reason led me to where I am today: sharing my hair growth experiences, knowledge and successes for you to read. This would not have happened for me if I wasn't willing to make the conscious decision to go against what I had been taught all my life about black hair growth and to discover things I never knew about caring for Afro hair.

I really hope the information contained within this book has been helpful. Ensure you refer back to it often to help keep you on track and I wish you the best of luck on your hair growth journey.

Further Reading

Books

Ultra Black Hair Growth II by Cathy Howse
Black Hair Growth Secrets Revealed by Elizabeth Vincent
The Afro Hair & Beauty Bible by Alison Husbands

Hair Care Forums

www.blackhairmedia.com
www.longhaircareforum.com

Information websites / References

www.julieoli.com
http://www.ehow.com
www.ezinearticles.com
www.healthyafrohair.com
www.hairinformation.com
http://www.elmhurst.edu/~chm/vchembook/184ph.html
http://www.livestrong.com/article/67204-biotin-thicken-hair/
http://www.hshairclinic.co.uk/hair-loss/all-about-hair/hair-cycle/
http://farbotanicals.com/hair-i-q/alcohol-is-bad-for-your-hair-right/
http://www.livecurlylivefree.blogspot.com/2009/01/hair-porosity.html
http://www.naturallycurly.com/curlreading/curl-products/curlchemist-porosity-and-curly-hair

Social media sites

YouTube
http://www.youtube.com/user/HealthyAfroHair

Twitter:
http://www.twitter.com/healthyafrohair

Facebook
http://www.facebook.com/healthyafrohair

Fokti:
http://www.public.fotki.com/healthyafrohair/

Flickr:
http://www.flickr.com/photos/healthyafrohair/

If you would like to get in contact regarding any of the information contained within this book, or you just have a general question, please feel free to reach me on the information below.

If you have a hair success story or a testimonial to share based on the methods you have applied within this book, please feel free to share it by sending me an email where you could possibly be featured on the website.

E: info@julieoli.com / info@healthyafrohair.com

W: www.julieoli.com / www.healthyafrohair.com